SAVE ME A SEAT BY THE DRUMMER

Growing up with disability,
lasagna, Elvis, and a myriad
of other afflictions

By Carmine J. Scarpa

ISBN: 978-1-4303-2826-1

Cover photo of Carmine J. Scarpa
Cover design by Carmine J. Scarpa

Published by Lulu.com

In memory of my mother and father

ACKNOWLEDGMENTS

I want to thank Nadine Scarpa and Mary Ann Murphy for their invaluable help in proofreading this book. Mary Ann should further be thanked for putting up with my endless questions about grammar. I also want to thank Yamilee Bazile for her support throughout the process.

Moreover, I want to acknowledge all those who are mentioned in the book, since, quite literally, I could not have done it without them.

A NOTE ON FORMAT

Each episode in this book contains at least one recollection of my childhood or youth. Additionally, some episodes contain comments and/or reflections.

The bold face type at the start of the episode denotes the original recollection while each additional recollection within the same episode starts on a new line and begins with the word "and."

Any comments and/or reflections upon a particular episode start on a new line and begin after a hyphen.

The scientific community is learning more each day about memory; that cerebral happening caused by the firing of millions of neutrons. Some scientists believe that, at times, we confuse and commingle fragments of memories, thereby creating new memories that have never occurred except in our brain. Others believe that before some memories can do us harm, our brain changes them into something that is more acceptable or, in some instances, something we cannot recall. Perhaps that is our safety valve - our security blanket. Apparently, though, we have little or no control over these neurological events and, although we should temper our beliefs accordingly, it would be unhealthy, or at least impractical, to maintain this uncertainty upon all we remember. Mindful of these prefatory remarks, and except for certain memories that I have chosen not to reveal, my recollections, comments, and reflections on my childhood and youth include . . .

large breasted ladies (many dressed in black) with deep dark cleavages
and wondering how far into their bodies that darkness went
and asking myself, "Do babies come out of those valleys?"
- Some Italian women, as a sign of mourning, wore black in

public for a year or more after the death of a loved one. Some of the more elderly wore it for the rest of their lives.

Josephine, the teenaged girl who lived in the apartment next door
and playing mother and child with her
and, after invariably misbehaving, being put across her lap for a hairbrush spanking
and her playful, but methodical manner
and Josephine being ever so watchful, so that no one would catch us playing our game
- I later learned that Josephine got married and had several children of her own.

Mrs. Davis wielding her wooden paddle at Saint Ann's Catholic School
and second-grade students standing in line nervously awaiting their turn over her knee
and Mrs. Davis sternly warning, "Don't hold on to the desk," as she applied three whacks for a first offense, six for a second, and nine for a third
- I don't remember anyone getting more than nine whacks (or Mrs. Davis spanking a girl), but I left school early that year to have surgery. Not early enough, however, to avoid catching three.

Mrs. Davis handing the paddle to the mother of an unruly student
and the mother, after a few seconds of apparent uncertainty, taking the paddle and spanking the boy very soundly in front of the entire class
and the boy crying long and loud
- It was probably the first time I experienced being embarrassed for someone else.

my last parochial school uniform
and transferring to the A. Harry Moore School in the third grade
      (a public school for the physically handicapped
         . . . disabled . . . impaired . . . physically challenged
         . . . differently abled?)
and my mother purchasing my new school clothes from Morris
      (the short Jewish man who came to our house offering
      clothes and other goods for sale)
and my mother paying Morris a little each week or so when he
      came by attempting to sell something else
and my mother also paying Mr. Hoffman, the life insurance agent,
      a little each month when he came to the door
and Mr. Hoffman walking with a limp, and always being out of
      breath as he reached our third-floor, walk-up, cold-water
      flat
- When my father died, we collected one thousand dollars plus
interest on a paid-in-full life insurance policy.

Morris ringing our bell
and running to the door and asking, "Who is it?"
and shouting to my mother (who had been severely hearing
      impaired since her youth), "Ma, it's the Jew guy!"
- There was no disrespect intended. Indeed, I had always
considered myself special in that I was a Catholic of Italian
descent with a Jewish Aunt and two Jewish cousins (the wife and
children of my father's brother Louis). I later learned that this
union between Italian and Jew was not so uncommon. Later still,
I joined in such a union when Nadine and I were married.

my mother telling me that, soon after my birth, I had surgery
      on my back to correct some sort of boney protrusion
and never being clear as to what was actually done, but having
      a scar on my lower back to show for it

my tonsils being removed
and my brother Ralph (eighteen years my elder) telling me that I
      was going to see a Shirley Temple movie while the doctor
      did the surgery
and having a vivid and frightening nightmare from the anesthesia
and Shirley not being in it

Ralph being called "Butch" and "Sonny"

my first surgery on my left leg and foot at age eight
and being very apprehensive about the prospect of getting
      anesthesia again
and kicking and yelling as the doctor put the mask over my face

**my second surgery on my left leg and foot about six months
      later**
and the doctor cautioning others in the operating room, "Watch
      this kid. He's going to be trouble"

**being with about seven other kids in the children's ward of
      the hospital**
and sliding ice cubes from our water pitchers along the floor and
      into the elevator just outside our ward door

Linda writing in my eighth-grade autograph book:

      Roses are red
      Violets are blue
      Whatever you do
      Don't marry a Jew

and my father's reaction, "What if your Aunt sees this?"
and his changing the word "Jew" to "stew"
and his reasoning being, "A stew is a drunk"
- I don't think my Aunt ever saw the book; however, if she did,
I'm fairly certain she wasn't fooled.

**Dell's entry in my autograph book (Dell and Donna were
    twins, very sexy, and about three years my elders):**

> The devil sends a naughty wind
> To blow the girls' skirts high
> But God in just, sends the dust
> To blind the bad man's eye

- Years later, while sitting in my car and checking the sights at
windy intersections, I would be sure to roll up my windows.

Donna's skirt
and lifting it up in Andy's candy store, as her boyfriend Bob
    encouraged me and held her arms
and my mother walking into the candy store at the end of one of
    those uplifting moments, just as Donna's skirt came to
    rest in the down position
- Whew!

**Bob, the oldest guy on the block, and his "radio bike" (a bike
    with a built-in radio)**
and Bob not being satisfied with it
and his anxiously awaiting his seventeenth birthday so he could
    buy a car

Bob's white Ford convertible
and sitting behind the steering wheel while it was parked outside
      Andy's

knowing all the makes, models, and years of cars
and that changing in the early 1960's when they all seemed to
      blend together
and my father's 1959 Chevy with the cat's eyes

**my brother Morris (fourteen years my elder) writing in my
      autograph book:**

      To a brother who is fatter than I
      Because he eats too much pizza pie

and Morris calling me "fat boy" (As Norton said to Kramden in
      the Honeymooners, "Maybe the phrase just fits")
and, since he was working and paying board, his complaining to
      our mother when she didn't have a "real meal" for him at
      supper
and our mother making him a "cubed" steak or some other
      culinary delight, while the rest of us ate hot dogs (or some
      similarly mundane fare)
and Morris, about an hour after finishing his "real meal,"
      shouting from the living room (or the parlor, as we called
      it), "Hey, fat boy! Tell mama to make me a hot dog!"
- My mother didn't actually make mundane fare very often. She
was an excellent cook. Indeed, too good.

Morris being called "Brother"
- He was actually baptized "Mauro." I guess that is Italian for
Morris. I have always called him Brother, as did most of our

family (including our mother and father). I would sometimes introduce him as my "brother Brother." At least one of our cousins calls him "Cousin Brother." His ex-wife Margie called him "Blackie," and our nieces and nephew call him "Uncle Moose." I'm sure, also, that he has been called some other names along the way.

holiday mornings
and getting up early due to the aroma of food throughout the
      house
and my mother laying the freshly made ravioli on the beds to dry
- Clean sheets were always used.

Sunday mornings
and rolling out of bed at about 10:30 a.m. and sitting down to a
      full dinner
- My father worked as a bartender on Sunday and started at noon.

my father making a cabinet and bookcase top for our stereo
      console out of an old discarded bed headboard
and my brothers and I laughing at him
and my father having the last laugh since the top turned out
      remarkably nice.

Lorraine being my first case of unrequited love
and the leg brace she wore due to Polio
and, at her request, buying her a twenty-five-cent Rock Hudson
      magazine
and giving it to her on the school bus the next day
and her promptly reporting me to her teacher
and being advised by her teacher the following year that, had it

not been for my poor deportment, I might have skipped a
grade
- To make matters worse, I could have gotten a soda, a bag of
potato chips, and quite a bit of penny candy with that quarter.

**Marion being my second case of unrequited love (Is there a
pattern developing here?)**
and her barely perceptible case of Cerebral Palsy
and how she first said she liked me and then said she didn't
and wanting to believe that her family discouraged the
relationship due to our age difference
- I was eleven and she was nine (although she had the body of a
twelve-year-old). Many years later, I saw her walking with
another young woman on a local college campus. I became
apprehensive at the thought of talking to her again, but my
anxiety was short-lived. Although we passed close enough to
have touched, neither of us acknowledged the other.
Contemporaneously with the writing of this recollection, I read in
a newspaper obituary that Marion's mother had died. Curious to
see how Marion looked more than thirty-five years after we first
rode together on the school bus, I parked my car outside the
church and waited for her to exit the funeral mass. I was
surprised, however, when she finally did. It was as if I were
looking at a computer-generated, age-enhanced version of the
picture stored in my mind's eye. I was not ready, willing, or able
to see the middle-aged woman standing before me. This person
was not Marion. Perhaps, too, I didn't want to think of the
middle-aged man I had become. Sometimes, it is certainly better
to leave well enough alone.

Mahatma Gandhi
and having been born the same year that the great man died
and thinking that perhaps I was Gandhi's reincarnate

and my best friend John Thiel saying to me, "If that's true, then
        Gandhi's soul has regressed"
- I think John may have actually said "digressed," but then we
were very young - and yes, John was my best friend.

vegetarianism
and how I abstained from eating meat for three months (John and
        Yoko were doing it, you know)
and stopping at a hot dog wagon and getting a weird look from
        the proprietor when I asked him for "onions on a bun"
and my longing for a White Castle hamburger finally getting the
        better of me
- I guess John was right. Gandhi could probably have withstood
such temptation.

Transcendental Meditation
and how John and I went to New York to speak to an Indian Guru
        about lessons, after having just seen The Beatles on TV
        touting the Maharishi Mahesh Yogi (The Maharishi was
        such a joyful person, always laughing and giggling as he
        spoke)
and the New York Guru, in the middle of teaching a class when
        we arrived, giving us some literature to read
and John's eyes momentarily straying from the materials
and the Guru, with fire in his eyes, screaming, "You are not
        reading!"
and John looking back at him as if to say, what's your problem,
        man?
- Needless to say, this pseudo holy man did not impress us, and
we did not take the classes. I remember hearing years later how
The Beatles became disillusioned with the Maharishi after
learning that he had been screwing some of the women in their
entourage.

playing in a band called the "Wanderers" with John, Sandy,
Guido, and Ricky

changing the band's name to The Forbidden Fruit
and then, Peck's Bad Boys
- Later on, when we started to play more adult nightclubs,
weddings, and such, we became The Front Page and, lastly, The
Mark Richards Orchestra. Although I stopped playing after I met
Nadine, the guys and I sometimes spoke about reuniting. That
thought ended when Sandy died.

the band auditioning for Bobby Blue
and Bobby being a booking agent and musician who had come to
        hear us
and Bobby having polio and walking with crutches
and my singing "Georgia on My Mind" for him
and his advising us that the key should be changed because it was
        too low for me
and the band members looking quizzically at each other since we
        had really never contemplated the idea of a key change
        (We just played whatever was printed on the music sheet)
and suddenly singing the song much stronger and brighter
- Many years later, after having retired "Georgia on My Mind"
from our repertoire, and while playing at the Union Club in
Hoboken, a very elderly woman came up to me while I was
singing and said, "I don't know much about music, but I know
what I like . . . " As I started to nod thank you, she continued,
". . . and you guys stink."

my father's "sayings," including "Your sister!" and "You
        remind me of my Uncle" or ". . . my Aunt"
and his teasing reply after being asked to go out somewhere,

"Yea, sure, I'll go. Save me a seat by the drummer" (the
event not necessarily being a musical one)
- I was never quite sure how this drummer "saying" came into
being. What was the nature of the drummer? Was a seat by the
drummer desirable or undesirable? My father did take me to see
"The Gene Krupa Story," starring Sal Mineo. I know, however,
from playing gigs with my band that most people don't care to sit
by the band, never mind the drummer. Yet the drummer is the
backbone, the pulse, the heartbeat of a band. Maybe it was the
ambiguity of the "saying," or more still its absurdity, that caught
my attention. Nevertheless, I am using these and other "sayings"
of my father more often as I get older.

**my father making groaning sounds when getting up from a
      chair**
and my inability to understand why he did that
- Now, I do it.

the "Sinatra Stories"
and how my father heard Sinatra sing at the Rustic Cabin in
      Englewood Cliffs, New Jersey (My father worked as a
      singing bartender, although I don't believe he ever
      worked at the Rustic Cabin)
and how Sinatra bought "coffee and . . ." for the locals at
      Bickfords Restaurant on Journal Square in Jersey City
and how my father and Barney Harvey (one of Sinatra's early
      piano accompanists) went to see "the voice" in his hotel
      room during an engagement at New York's Paramount
      Theater
and how, upon leaving the hotel room, the three of them were
      mobbed by a group of "bobby-soxers" (I'm sure they
      were not after Barney or my father)
and how Sinatra gave my father an autographed picture that day

- Although I thought that my father may have had a hand in personalizing the photo, I never wanted to put him on the spot by asking him about it. Due to my uncertainty, though, I rarely showed the photo. Just recently, however, a friend of the family asked me, "Wasn't your father once with Sinatra when 'bobby-soxers' mobbed them?" He had heard the story some twenty-five years earlier. I nodded and thought to myself: Perhaps I should begin carrying a few wallet-sizes of that photo. Many years later, I purchased an original photograph of Sinatra from photographer Sammy Siegel. I had viewed his work at an Exhibit on Long Island where he also showed pictures of other personalities, including Judy Garland, The Beatles, and Richard Nixon. I picked up the picture at Sammy Siegel's house after the exhibit came down. While there, I noticed a picture of Sammy Siegel with Sinatra hanging on the living room wall. Mrs. Siegel saw me looking at the photograph and remarked, "Sammy took that picture." With a quizzical look on my face, I said, "Sammy?" She said, "Yes, Sammy Davis, Jr."

Susan sitting in front of me in Mrs. Davidson's third-grade classroom
and how she was recovering from a broken leg or some other
        orthopedic problem
and how around midyear, she began to walk without her crutches
and shortly thereafter, Susan telling us that she was going back to
        her "normal" school
and the day her skirt got caught on the back of her chair as she sat
        down
and staring at her white panties all during arithmetic
- Although Susan, at such a tender age, may not have had very much of a figure, it was much more interesting than those being posted on the blackboard by Mrs. Davidson.

the grammar school bathroom being called the "lavatory"

**the day an unpleasant odor pervaded the third-grade
     classroom**
and being red-faced with embarrassment, since it was obvious
          that the odor was most pronounced around my desk
and Mrs. Davidson saying to me, "Go to the lavatory and see if
          it's you" (Did she really believe that if it was me, that I
          didn't already know it?)
and sitting on the toilet and hearing someone come into the room
          and enter the stall next to mine
and knowing from his shoes that it was Mr. Bruno, the morbidly
          obese man who assisted the more severely disabled
          children
and staring at his feet and noticing how one rose up and
          disappeared from my view
and watching as the other foot rose up and also disappeared
and knowing that if I were to look up toward the top of the next
          stall, I would see Mr. Bruno's face spying down at me
- Needless to say, I was sent home early that day.

my truancy in high school
and its origin in grammar school when I would chew a mouthful
          of cookies, spit them into the toilet bowl, and tell my
          mother that I had thrown up (Chocolate chips seemed to
          have the best mix of color and texture)
and then watching "I Love Lucy," "Abbott and Costello," and the
          folks from Mayberry on TV, while eating my mother's
          fine cooking
- My mother never seemed bewildered by my swift recoveries. I
would be vomiting at seven and feasting by eight. Perhaps she
liked the company. I know she liked to see me eat. It was cute,
back then, for a little kid to be chubby. I was one hundred and

ninety-eight pounds in the eighth grade. A real cutie-pie.

quitting high school
and being absent so many days (89, I think) that the principal
      gave me an ultimatum: "Come to school everyday for
      these last two months of the year, or you won't graduate"
and taking off two days the very next week
- I was one of two high school dropouts in my law school
graduating class.

selling light bulbs by telephone at a not-for-profit company
      that employed only the disabled
and leaving that job before selling one bulb
- I later got a high school equivalency diploma and began Saint
Peter's College in the evening as a Political Science major.
Within a year, I transferred to the day session as pre-med
(spending so much time at the podiatrist, I thought why not
become one), then switched to Theology, then Sociology, before
finally graduating as an Art History major.

eighth-grade graduation rehearsals
and the class being seated on stage according to size
and being seated up front since I was short
and a teacher remarking that perhaps I should be seated toward
      the back
and another teacher countering, "But Carmine sits short"
and the former teacher answering, "Yes, but Carmine also sits
      wide"
- We didn't have the traditional walk-up-on-stage-to-receive-
your-diploma procession since, in a school for the disabled, it
would have been time prohibitive.

Frankie being a new kid on the block
and his laughing when I told him I went to A. Harry Moore
and his remarking, "You're kidding me. That school is for
         retards"
- Although we had no mentally impaired children at A. Harry
Moore, the physical limitations of some students may have made
the rate of learning slower than in other schools. Some severally
disabled students had difficulty speaking, turning pages, and even
holding up their heads. Not having any such difficulties, I got
good grades without expending very much effort. This study
habit still haunts me today.

Spina Bifida
and learning that this congenital, mobility-impairing disability
         involved a lack of fusion at the base of the spinal column
         (So maybe not in those exact words)
and thinking why, out of all the kids born into this world, did I
         have to be one of those born with this disease?
and not coming up with a good answer
- As an adult, I would realize that we all have our burdens to
bear. Some may be more inherently problematic than others, but
it's likely that we each expend just as much effort no matter what
our particular burden. A beauty queen worries as much about the
zit that might appear on her nose, as the police officer worries
about the bullet that might penetrate his chest.

**my mother warning me not to draw with ink on my skin
         because I would get blood poisoning**

**my mother not allowing the barber to give me the D.A.
         (Duck's Ass) haircut I wanted**

clothes
and admiring the way other kids dressed
- Often, by the time I got the same or similar item, it was out of
style. I used to like the bell-bottomed trousers worn by the black
guys at Snyder High School. Fortunately, or unfortunately as the
case may be, coupling my large waist size with my short inseam,
all of my trousers looked like bell-bottoms.

Pesin's - the clothing store
and being led downstairs to the "husky" section when shopping
        for my Easter suit

Bruce
and how I always lost when we wrestled
and arguing that it would be different if we were on equal footing
and getting on our knees to compensate for my lack of leg
        strength and balance
and losing the "knees" matches also

**selling Sunday newspapers (on Saturday evening) with Bruce
        in Jersey City**
and having my own corner
and finding fewer and fewer papers each time I returned from
        using the corner tavern's bathroom
and the wind blowing some of the remaining papers all around
        the sidewalk
- I think I cleared about thirty-five cents that night.

Bruce and I playing spin the bottle with Kathy
and, when the opportunity to kiss her arose, shaking hands
        instead

Bruce's father, an evangelical minister, saying to me,
    "Someday I'm going to take you to a place where a
    man will heal you without the use of a knife"
and not quite understanding the concept, but eventually going
    with Bruce and his parents to a big assembly hall in
    Newark, New Jersey
and enjoying the spirited gospel singing of an all black choir
and getting in a long line and walking toward the front of the hall
and the minister, who had been preaching, stopping to put his
    hand on my head, and saying some words which I don't
    recall
and getting back to my seat and hearing Bruce ask his father for
    some money so that he and I could get Chinese food from
    the take-out across the street
-Many years later, I read in a local newspaper that Bruce and his
brother had been arrested. They were accused of kidnapping a
young woman, and holding her captive in an apartment for
several days while repeatedly raping and sodomizing her.

ordering pizza to the houses of guys we didn't like
and the time that one of the parents actually took the pie

my friend Al
and first meeting him in my late teens when he was on leave
    from the Navy
and Al purchasing an old junk heap of a car during each leave
    (paying about $50.00 or so)
and greatly enjoying Al's leaves, since riding with him gave me a
    feeling of mobility and freedom
- Even today, you might say I am symbiotically attached to my
car.

17

the time Al farted in the balcony of a large and nearly empty movie theater
and how it echoed
and my friends and I having a prolonged fit of giggling
- The same thing happened to me with another friend years later in church, only I was the culprit. My friend and I could never again sit in the same pew without laughing hysterically. Did I say "pew?"

Sandy (the drummer in our band) farting in a crowded car
and the driver, another band member's father, opening the car door to get air as he drove down the highway

John and I keeping count of our farts
and having a new contest each evening

John's brother, Tommy, telling me that John had wanted to be a priest until he met me

Tommy calling me "Duke" (He actually called me the "Duke of Ellington")
and the nickname catching on with musician friends
and listing "Duke" as my nickname in the Local 526 American Federation of Musicians' Union Directory

taking my driver's test at age 17 in Sandy's father's Rambler station wagon (the Green Turtle) at Roosevelt Stadium in Jersey City

**Linda and I playing "show and tell" in the backyard of the
    abandoned laundry**

the dead cat
and dragging it to the abandoned laundry in a cardboard box
and telling my friends that I was going to bring it back to life (I
        had just seen the original Frankenstein movie on TV)
and eventually deciding that the task was too demanding for a
        person of my age, knowledge, and skill level
and my friends understanding all too well

my medical school
and having two students enroll against their better judgment
and asking them to copy a drawing that I had made of a heart
and their failing to submit the assignment and, consequently,
        never having a graduating class

wanting to be many things when I grew up

        a doctor - one of my doctors had given me a surgical
        mask. I used to put it on before making incisions in my
        Jerry Mahoney ventriloquist dummy. After removing
        some of Jerry's stuffing, I would sew him up with my
        mother's needle and thread

        a priest - I once had a faux altar set up in the living room.
        I would sit there and pray while my mother and father
        watched Milton Berle

        Elvis - I had nearly perfected the nose twitch and lip curl

        a lawyer - I used to watch Perry Mason and The

Defenders on TV. (Does anybody know why the
Defenders has never been shown in reruns?)

- As it turned out, after working in a fork lift rental office for a
year after college, and then spending several years as a
commercial artist, I did become a lawyer. I wish now that I had
thought more seriously about becoming Elvis.

**my brother Ralph taking me to see Elvis' first movie "Love
Me Tender" at the State Theater on Journal Square**
and having a heavy plaster cast covering my left leg due to
        surgery
and having a strong urge to go to the bathroom during the movie
and not wanting to climb the long flight of stairs on crutches
        (Perhaps, more importantly, not wanting to miss any of
        the movie)
and Elvis dying at the end of the movie
- To this day, at anyone's mention of "Love Me Tender," Ralph
will remind me of how I killed Elvis by "shitting my pants."

the New York premiere of "Love Me Tender"
and seeing the newspaper advertisement for it
and it being a full-page ad with a picture of Elvis playing his
        guitar
and going nuts believing that Elvis was going to be there in
        person
and crying and carrying on because no one would take me to see
        him
- Up to that time, Elvis had only been a sound on record and an
image on TV. Suddenly he was real. They didn't understand how
important this was to me. I finally did get to see Elvis in person
some twenty-five years later at New York's Madison Square
Garden. He died (for real) about five years after that

performance. Somewhat ironically, he died on his bathroom floor.

Confirmation
and wanting to take "Elvis" as my confirmation name
and my parents saying no because it would be insulting to my
      brother Ralph who was my sponsor
- Does anyone ever use a confirmation name?

**my father and I arguing over who was better, Elvis or
      Sinatra**
- Although some years later I would agree with my father that
Sinatra was one of the greatest singers of all time, I don't recall
my father ever acknowledging Elvis' abilities so clearly. My
father died just two months before Elvis. When I first heard of
Elvis' death, my initial reaction was to wonder what my father
would say when he heard the news. That was probably the
moment I first realized that my father was no longer there for me.

**telling my third-grade teacher that I played the guitar
      and sang**
and actually having a guitar, but not knowing how to play it
and always singing with my father and brother Ralph
and even harmonizing with Ralph on "Dear Old Dad"
and the third-grade teacher asking me to bring in my guitar so I
      could perform for her and another teacher
and Ralph, when learning of my problem, telling me to tap on the
      guitar while singing
and finally singing "Can't You Tell That I'm in Love with You"
      for the teachers while tapping away on my guitar
and later that afternoon, with my guitar in position, and while
      standing in front of the entire third-grade class, putting

my arm straight out toward the audience (à la Elvis) and
          singing the line: "Well it's one for the money"
and then suddenly freezing up and standing motionless and mute
          for what seemed to be an eternity before running into the
          clothing room
- After doing an internet search for the song, "Can't You Tell
That I'm in Love with You," and not finding it, I asked my
brother Ralph about the song. He remembered that my father
used to sing it, and that it was written by my father's friend,
Barney Harvey. It's possible that the song was never published.
Imagine, I was singing original material at such a young age.

watching a drama called "The Singing Idol" starring Tommy Sands on Kraft Theater in 1957

- Albeit, remembering that arguably first-ever rock 'n roll drama
as being "The Teenage Idol" on Playhouse 90.

Frankie Avalon, Bobby Rydell and, of course, Fabian

Rosemary

and asking her for a date (She lived a half block from me and
          went to A. Harry Moore apparently due to a heart
          condition)
and Rosemary being in the eighth grade (one year ahead of me)
and calling her on the telephone and pretending to be someone
          else
and telling her that a friend of mine, Carmine, liked her and
          wanted to know if she would go out on a date with him
and Rosemary immediately answering, "No"
and confessing my identity to her and resubmitting the question
and again her answering, "No"
- Except for a "date" with Mary at an ice cream parlor (Bruce

being there for moral support), I didn't traditionally "date" until law school. I always believed that my late blooming was due to my disability. And it was - but it was my perception of myself as a disabled person that held me back, and not the disability itself. I guess it was easier to believe that my disability was the problem, rather than looking to something that I had more control over.

reading aloud in parochial school
and standing in line around the perimeter of the classroom until it
         was my turn to read
and students being ridiculed by the teacher and laughed at by
         fellow students for making mistakes
- I don't remember ever being ridiculed or laughed at, but I do recall the stress of the situation. To this day, I get tense when I have to read aloud (or do anything in front of a crowd). I have never really enjoyed reading as a pastime.

**my mother crocheting doilies, tablecloths, bedspreads and
         other items while my father watched baseball on TV**
- She was truly expert at this craft. Almost everyone in our family (and outside our family) wanted one or more of her pieces. I keep one of my mother's doilies on the chest of drawers in my bedroom.

my mother saving plaid stamps
and green stamps
and getting dish sets (a piece or so each week) at the A & P

the nun dolls
- My mother told me that as a young child I would cry every time I saw a nun. Since she was planning to send me to parochial

school, my Aunt Tessie gave me a couple of nun dolls. (I remember comedian Pat Cooper once saying that every Italian family had an Aunt Tessie.) My aunt excelled at sewing and had made the nuns' habits. It must have worked because I was not frightened of nuns by the time I entered school. That changed, however, the first time I saw Sister Ann slam a kid's head into a blackboard.

my mother escorting me the two blocks to kindergarten
and the morning I was caught misbehaving in the schoolyard
      before class
and how the nun made me stand with my back to a concrete
      column and my hands stretched high into the air
and my mother's face as she watched
and my feeling bad for her because she was feeling bad for me
- Perhaps this was intended to calm me down, or perhaps it was to be my introduction to the crucifixion.

that same nun forcing me to spank myself with two drum
      sticks, for doing God-knows-what-awful-thing in
      kindergarten
and, reacting to my tears, a classmate caught my eye and advised
      me to hit myself softly
- He had not yet learned the difference between physical and psychological pain.

eating paste
- It was so tasty, too.

First Holy Communion
and the day we were rehearsing

and one girl repeatedly and frantically raising her hand asking to
go to the bathroom
and how the nuns just ignored her
and how she finally peed all over the floor
and how an angry nun grabbed the young girl, who was already
crying from embarrassment, bent her over, and spanked
her very hard as the entire group of cummunicants-to-be
watched

hearing that there was an eighth-grade spanking machine

spanking a few of the girls in the neighborhood
and being playful, but methodical
and my being ever so watchful, so that no one would catch us
playing our game
-We are all conditioned by our past. I don't believe, however, as
some people, that this "cause and effect" concept is limiting. I
think it should be viewed as positive and unifying in that all of
us, and all things, are inexorably linked. Perhaps, however, this
was not the best recollection on which to be philosophical.

the day I stole a religious medallion from a girl in first grade
and the nun finding it in my desk and slapping me across the face
and my telling the nun that the boy next to me gave it to me to
hold
and the nun sending both of us to the principal's office
and the principal, not being able to decide which one of us was
telling the truth, saying, "I'll leave it up to God to punish
the guilty party"
and often thinking of this episode when having a particularly bad
day
- I no longer view God as simply an old man in the sky who

rewards and punishes. I have intuited a more Kabbalistic view of God as everything - the infinite - the Ein Sof. This concept supports the wonderful idea that all of us, and all things, are connected. It further leaves intact that all-important mystery as to the ultimate nature of God, since we cannot expect to comprehend the infinite.

making confession and saying penance the evening before my surgery at twelve years old

watching the Sunday evening Judy Garland Show on television from my hospital room in the children's wing
- Since I had a private room and was a bit older than most of the other kids in the wing, the nurses would bend the rules a bit for me. What better antidote for recovery, though, than the last segment of that show with Judy singing her heart out amid the runway lights. Bravo to Peter Allen who would write and sing many years later, "Quiet Please, There's a Lady on Stage."

Aunt Dot and Uncle Lou bringing me an oil painting kit while I was in the hospital

taking special art classes at A. Harry Moore
and thinking about going to Paris one day to study art
- I have been to Paris twice as an adult (the first time on my honeymoon), but I have not become "une artiste Parisienne." The closest I came, was having one of my paintings accepted for an exhibit called "American Painters in Paris." I did not, however, participate in the show because I did not have the required entry fee or air fare for transporting the painting to Paris. As it turned

out, it was no real loss, since a few years later I read in an art magazine that the show had been predominantly a moneymaking venture. I have had some complimentary things said about my art work, however, including a teacher at New York City's School of Visual Arts saying that one of my class assignments was the best student art work he had seen that term. I still have thoughts about being a painter; however, I do more "thinking" than "doing." In this regard, I believe Descartes once said: "To do is to be." Or, was it Sartre who said: "To be is to do." Or, then again, was it Sinatra who said: "Do be do be do." (Sorry, it's an old one, but I couldn't resist.) The arts, however, have always been important to me. I believe that all acts are eternal acts in that they will influence all things forever. An artist's creation, being non-utilitarian, is a celebration of such influences.

looking at graphic pictures of holocaust victims in a book at my Aunt Dot's house
- I didn't know it at the time; but the disabled, too, fell victim to Hitler's notion of Aryan supremacy, although certainly not in any way comparable to the gargantuan atrocities committed against the Jews.

the "facts of life"
and being with Ralph and his wife Janet and asking my mother to
explain them
and my mother answering, by giving me a quick light slap across
the face
and Ralph and Janet laughing hysterically

Chuckie finally explaining the "facts of life" to me during sixth-grade lunch
and listening in disbelief and thinking, no wonder my mother

slapped me

my mother and her sisters singing "Melancholy Baby"

the kids playing "Buck Buck"
and one kid jumping on another's back
and then other kids jumping on one by one until everyone fell
      down
and not playing because I couldn't jump

the day J.F.K. was shot
and how, as we rode home on the school bus that afternoon, Mr.
      Brody, a six-foot, three-hundred pound, tough-as-nails-
      sort-of-guy, while holding a tiny transistor radio to his
      ear, turned to me with tears in his eyes and said, "He's
      dead"

missing the live telecast of Ruby shooting Oswald, but
      catching the first replay moments later

cheering along with other kids as a car rode through the
      streets advising that, due to the funeral of J.F.K.,
      there would be no school on Monday

the Cuban Missile Crisis
and J.F.K. speaking to the nation on TV
and the next morning in class, waiting patiently with fellow
      students for the bomb to drop
and being slightly disappointed when nothing happened

air raid drills
and having to get under our desks in parochial school
- At A. Harry Moore, most of the kids couldn't get under their desks; so instead we were marched into a room near the center of the building. This room was not likely a fallout shelter, but it was free of windows. I guess the thinking was that students would not be hurt by flying glass when the big one fell.

thinking about working on Bobby Kennedy's presidential primary campaign in New Jersey
and watching Bobby's late night victory speech in the California Primary on TV
and waking the next morning, to learn that Bobby had been assassinated just minutes after he concluded that victory speech
- He was assassinated just twenty-five days before my twentieth birthday - a significant marker for the end of my teenage years.

having trouble keeping up with the rest of the class, as we would line up and march into parochial school each morning and afternoon to Sousa's "Stars and Stripes Forever"

my mother telling me that, as a baby, I was slow to walk
and how she brought me to the doctor who delivered me
and the doctor saying, "Madam, you should be happy that the army will never take your son"
and how my mother angrily replied, "Doctor, I wish my son were healthy so that the army would want to take him"
- Perhaps every cloud does have a silver lining.

**my father telling me that when I turned sixteen I would have
    an operation that would correct my disability**
and talking about this from time to time as I grew up
- By the time I neared sixteen, however, my father was no longer
telling me this and I was no longer asking him about it.

**overhearing Uncle Al (Aunt Tessie's husband) saying to my
    father that the doctor should cut my foot off and give
    me a wooden one**
and asking my father about it later that night
and my father telling me that he wanted to punch my uncle for
    saying that

hearing my father praying each night before he went to sleep

**my father taking my mother and me to see Anthony Newley
    in "The Roar of the Greasepaint, the Smell of the
    Crowd" on Broadway for our birthdays (I was the 1st
    of July, and my mother was the 4th of July)**
and the orchestra seats costing $6.25
and the show being more for me than for my mother, since I was
    the Anthony Newley fan
and my mother sleeping through much of the show (Her hearing
    impairment made it difficult for her to hear the show
    properly, and I guess she became bored)
and going to "The Jade," a fancy Chinese restaurant on Journal
    Square, after the show
and my father being so proud because he was able to pronounce
    "Moo Goo Gai Pan"

Frankie (a second one) being the neighborhood bully
and finally believing that I could "take" him
and purposely throwing a football at his head to provoke a fight
and actually making his mouth bleed before he "gave"
- No, I wasn't hoisted on everyone's shoulders, but my friends
were very happy because Frankie no longer bothered us.

Frankie's mother working for Thumans (the meat products
        manufacturer)
and how she would periodically make hot dogs for all of us
and how she passed them out of her ground floor window

the telephone exchange "656" replacing "Oldfield 6"
and "332" replacing "Delaware 2"
and "434" replacing "Henderson 4"
and "795" replacing "Swathmore 5"

dialing 411 for telephone information
and cursing at the information lady (They were all ladies at the
        time)
and then begging her not to tell my mother, as she persistently
        rang back our number asking to speak to an adult
and how she finally agreed to let me off the hook, after I
        apologized and promised never to do it again
and my mother asking me what was going on when she saw me
        repeatedly answering the phone
and telling her that it was a friend playing a joke

our telephone party line
and picking up the receiver and shouting something rude (I guess
        I didn't learn my lesson)

31

and being very surprised when the voice at the other end said
very authoritatively, "You'd better stop, Scarpa, or I'll tell
your brother!"
- No one had told me that we shared a party line with a police
officer friend of my brother Morris.

my mother's first hearing aid
and coming home from school that first day and knocking on the
door
and knowing something was different when my mother
immediately answered the door (I would sometimes have
to pound quite a few times)
and being very happy for my mother, but also realizing that I
wouldn't be getting away with as much anymore
- I think that we all act in our own "self-interest." But I don't see
this as necessarily negative. Even stepping in front of a loved one
to take a bullet is an act of "self-interest" because the potential
consequences of not doing so - seeing the loved one die - can be
more adverse to our well-being than taking the bullet ourselves.
The negativity enters when our "self-interest" is completely
devoid of the interest of others.

**how Rockefeller's money couldn't buy better coffee than
Chock Full O' Nuts**

how Carter had little "liver" pills

**watching "Mighty Joe Young" and "The People Against
O'Hara" (with Spencer Tracy) over and over again,
all week on the Million Dollar Movie**

**watching John Wayne and Robert Stack safely bring their
jetliner home in "The High and the Mighty" (over and
over again)**
and John Wayne whistling the theme song as he walked away
from the plane at the end of the movie

**being infatuated with Teresa Wright in "Pride of the
Yankees"**
and with Ingrid Bergman in "The Bells of St. Mary's"

Debbie Reynolds singing "Tammy"
and Richard Chamberlain singing "Three Stars Will Shine
Tonight" (the theme song from the Doctor Kildare
television show)

"Ben Casey," "Ben Casey," "Ben Casey"

watching "Winky Dink and You" on TV
and putting a plastic sheet over the screen so that I could draw on
the TV, when prompted by the show's host
- You would be asked to draw a ladder or some other item to help
Winky get out of a jam.

**putting a tri-colored plastic sheet over the TV screen to
simulate color TV**

being one of the first in the neighborhood to get a color TV
and "Bonanza" being the first color show my family (and
friends) watched

going to the hospital by ambulance, after cutting my arm trying to fly through a glass door while playing "Superman"

putting "Pop Beads" on Buttons (my black cat)
and my friends and relatives fearing Buttons because he scratched

watching Liberace and Jimmy Durante on TV
- "I'll Be Seeing You" and "Young at Heart" will always carry special meanings for me.

waiting for Jerry Lewis to cry each year, at the end of his telethon when singing "You'll Never Walk Alone"

Judy Garland's rendition of "Smile" (the song Jerry Lewis used as his theme)
- Later learning that "Smile" was written by Charlie Chaplain.

Sam Levenson and Myron Cohen

John and I watching the Donna Reed Show on TV and ogling Shelley Fabares in a pair of tight white shorts
and my purchasing her recording of "Johnny Angel"
and my not purchasing Paul Peterson's "My Dad" (although it was a pleasant recording)

seeing the movie "Inherit the Wind"
and "Compulsion"
and "Where the Boys Are"
and "Rodan"
and "Godzilla"
and "Rebel Without a Cause"

watching "Superman" on TV
and "I Married Joan"
and "The Life of Riley"
and "Ozzie and Harriet"
and "Make Room for Daddy"
and "Abbott and Costello"
and "The Jackie Gleason Show" (with "The Honeymooners")
and "The Mickey Mouse Club" (with the letters on Annette's
    shirt getting harder to read each year).

enjoying Johnny Ray's singing on the Ed Sullivan Show
and how he started ripping off his clothes as he sang

the Mills Brothers singing "Paper Doll" and "Glow Worm"

Mr. Blue by The Fleetwoods

**John Seccafico giving a speech in class about his favorite
    television shows**
and how he purposely said "Dick Van Dyke" and "Alfred
    Hitchcock" with heavy accents on the "Dick" and the
    "cock"
and his believing that he was putting one over on the teacher

debating John Seccafico on slavery in front of our fifth-grade class

and being so proud after writing my closing speech that I
couldn't help but read it to John before the debate

and John telling me how good it was

and John, going first in the debate, purposely using all of my
words in his speech and making it impossible for me to
then use my own words without sounding ridiculous

being a safety patrol officer on the school bus

and wearing one of those white belts that went around the waist
and diagonally across the chest

**my father having to go to school because I was caught
carrying a paperback book based on The
Untouchables TV show**

and the principal telling my father that I shouldn't be watching
shows like The Untouchables

and my father letting me watch it the next time it was on but
cautioning me not to tell anyone at school

lasagna being one of my favorite foods

and ravioli

and manicotti

and breaded veal cutlet

and corn (with lots of butter and salt)

**calling spaghetti "pissghetti," pretzels "bretzels," and pizza
"bizza"**

Aunt Tessie's homemade bizza

my mother's chicken soup

one of my favorite toys being a Colt 45, with a cylinder that popped out and bullets with removable shells
and many doctor kits
and Indian feathers
and the Robin Hood castle (with working catapult) that my
      brother Ralph bought me upon my coming home from the
      hospital at age eight

Ralph telling me that he would ask Father Rigney to make me an altar boy when I became of age
and my no longer being interested after being transferred to A.
      Harry Moore

Ralph taking me to see Zippy the Chimp at the Jersey City Armory

going to see the Three Stooges at the Stanley Theater on Journal Square
and Officer Joe Bolton being there to introduce them
and how the side walls of the Stanley were designed with Roman
      style architectural elements
and the ceiling being painted to simulate sky with lights for stars
- I also saw the live closed-circuit showing of the first Ali-Frazier
heavyweight championship fight at the Stanley with my father
and Sandy. The building today is owned and used as an assembly
hall by The Jehovah's Witnesses.

the Loew's Theater on Journal Square with its elaborate Art Deco lobby and balcony (We called it the "Lowees")

John and I going to his high school (St. Aloysius) for a basketball game
and leaving at half-time and taking the "Tubes" to New York (The Hudson-Manhattan Tubes is now the PATH train)
and getting to New York, taking the escalator to street level (at 33rd), looking at the snow falling on the city street, and going home
and of course telling our parents that the game was great (Sure glad they didn't ask who won)

John and I wearing our trench coat linings (without the coat, of course) as a fashion statement (after seeing someone else do it first)

not going to the dentist until age seventeen
and finally making an appointment at the dental school in Jersey City
and being so frightened that my legs were shaking as I sat in the chair
and their sending me home with a prescription for Valium to be taken prior to my next visit
and it not being much different the next time, when the student began cleaning my teeth manually (with the "pick" tool)
and it sounding as if my teeth were cracking
and telling him to stop and that I would not be returning
- I didn't visit a dentist again until a few years later when I had seventeen cavities filled. Although my teeth were (and are still) somewhat crooked, I was fortunate that except for the cavities, they were healthy. I considered braces when I was about thirty,

but thought about it taking two years or so and decided not to invest the time (I still was not too thrilled with dentists either). My brother Morris once said to me when I was considering not going to law school because of the time involved, that the time will pass anyway, so the only difference will be whether you get there with or without the degree.

working behind the counter at Andy's candy store (unpaid, of course)
and sneaking a piece of penny candy now and then when Andy
     went to the bathroom

Nana and Pap Pap (our elderly and old-worldly Italian landlords at 1085 Summit Avenue in Jersey City - where I lived from my birth in 1948 until my father had his first heart attack in 1970)
and their being like grandparents to me
and watching Pap Pap put snuff up his nose
and watching Pap Pap sneeze
and watching the snails that Pap Pap used to let crawl around in
     the backyard
and finding out that those snails would eventually make their way
     into Nana's Sunday gravy (a.k.a., tomato sauce)
- Years later, I began eating those little creatures when Nadine
and I ordered them in France: "Les escargots, s'il vous plait."

Playing chess with Pap Pap
- I learned later that we weren't actually playing chess. We were using the chess pieces to play checkers. No wonder a pawn was able to jump a queen.

**going into Nana and Pap Pap's for a drink of water, instead
of climbing the two flights of stairs to our apartment
(They lived in a house which was separate from our
building)**
and Pap Pap dying
and a large gathering of people coming to see Nana
and my mother telling me to say, "Sorry for your troubles," if
I went in for a drink
and everyone being very quiet when I finally did go in
and my saying, "Nana, sorry for your troubles"
and all of a sudden, several old women dressed in black
(including Nana) starting to scream and cry hysterically
- I went dry for the rest of the summer.

**knowing only one of my grandparents (my paternal
grandmother)**
and never even seeing a picture of my maternal grandfather who
died at a very young age

being a page boy at my cousin Mary's wedding to Matty
and wearing a white tuxedo jacket
and my cousin Florence being a flower girl

**"That Old Black Magic," with my cousin Andrew mimicking
Louis Prima to his first wife's Keely Smith**

**visiting my Aunt Dot and Uncle Lou (and their big
backyard) in Rutherford, New Jersey**
and singing "Twilight Time" with my cousin Marilyn
and my cousin Ralph with his electric trains
- Although Rutherford was only about twenty minutes by car

from Jersey City, it felt like a trip to the country.

**My Aunt Mamie having an "in-ground" pool in Rahway,
        New Jersey**
and my Uncle Tony (with my cousins Tony and Bill) building his
        own house
and my cousin Loretta liking Pat Boone better than Elvis
and my cousin Gerard always talking about "Campy" (Roy
        Campanella)
- Rahway was really the country in those days.

Bobby Darin
and my mother and her sisters thinking that we might be related
        to him because their maiden name was "Cassotta" and his
        real name was "Walden Robert Cassotto"
- Close (seven out of eight letters).

my Aunt Mary yelling at my cousin Joe
and my father always calling Joe, "Giuseppe"
- I call him that also.

my Aunt Rose calling me "Tom"
- My father used the name, "Tommy," when he sang. His given
name was Carmine. I am a junior, but discontinued using it after
my father died.

**celebrating Christmas and New Year's Eves with my
        grandmother, aunts and uncles, and cousins**
and Uncle Al playing Santa one year
and my yelling out, "Hey, I know those shoes. You're Uncle Al!"

41

- I remember a veritable banquet of fish and seafood. Unfortunately, I didn't like fish and seafood at the time. I wish now that I had those days back (and not only for the food). Happily, a few years ago, at my Cousin Florence's urging, many of us cousins (on my father's side) began getting together several times a year.

Christmases at 1085 Summit Avenue
and the smell of a real tree
and long strands of silver tinsel
and searching endlessly for that one burned-out light bulb
and my feet getting cold from walking on a linoleum covered
        floor
and Lionel and American Flyer trains
and a fire truck with a working ladder
and sleeping on the couch attempting to catch Santa
and having milk and cookies for Santa and carrots for the
        reindeer (There were probably a few goodies for me, too)
- I don't remember many Christmases after leaving 1085 Summit Avenue.

**adorning my accordion lesson books with the ski patches that
        came on jars of Ovaltine drink mix**

**my father purchasing my first accordion from my godfather,
        Joe (Small) Romanelli, and giving it to me as a
        Christmas surprise**
and Joe taking "numbers" in a little candy store which he
        operated solely for that purpose
and the store having a refrigerator with a few bottles of soda and
        a glass case with some candy bars
and Joe practically chasing the kids away when they came in to

purchase something

and Joe playing accordion and piano by ear (not with his hands? - ta dum!)

and my taking accordion lessons for about four years until the British Rock Invasion came along and, alas, the accordion was no longer the instrument of choice (not even for a chubby Italian kid)

and my father not being happy about my wanting to switch to guitar, but finally allowing me to stop accordion lessons

and my father buying me a Silvertone electric guitar (a brand made for Sears & Roebuck) with an amplifier built into the guitar case

arguing with my father about how he was wasting his money playing "numbers"

and my father purchasing all of my future instruments from money he made from "hitting the numbers"

- How hypocritical of me, telling my father that he was wasting his money playing "numbers" when I gladly became the major recipient of the fruits of such activity. Sometimes acknowledging a memory can be helpful.

my father purchasing a pearl ring as a birthday gift for my mother

and how my mother loved that ring

my father purchasing a sapphire ring for himself

- After he died, I began wearing that ring.

my father being a Brooklyn Dodger fan

and how he used to tell me about the games he saw at Ebbets

Field
and how he later abandoned the "Bums" (after they abandoned
        Brooklyn) and became a Mets fan

my father being a Yankee hater (I was a Yankee fan)
and how he would love to say, when the opportunity presented
        itself, "Hey, the Yankees won. Detroit had six"
- My father wanted me to think "won," but of course, he meant
"one."

**my father telling me about the boxing matches he saw at the
        Jersey City Gardens**
and the time he saw Dempsey fight at "Boyle's Thirty Acres" in
        Jersey City
and his taking me to see Rubin "Hurricane" Carter at the "old"
        Madison Square Garden
- None of the above remain standing (except for "Hurricane").

my father and I watching the Friday Night Fights
and seeing Benny (The Kid) Paret knocked out by Emile Griffith
and Paret dying some days later

**my father taking me to see a minor league baseball game at
        Roosevelt Stadium in 1961**
and hearing over the public address system that Roger Maris had
        hit home runs 37, 38, 39, and 40 during a
        twi-night doubleheader at Yankee Stadium
and the infielders making numerous errors in one inning
and the manager coming out to the mound to change the pitcher
and someone in the stands yelling, "Hey, don't change the
        pitcher, change the infield"

44

**my final childhood surgery at age twelve (on my right leg
     and foot)**
and being carried up two flights of stairs on the back of the
          owner of the corner tavern, on my return home from the
          hospital
- The surgeries were performed to allow me to walk with my feet
flat to the ground. Until that time, I was walking on the balls of
my feet. The downside of the surgeries was that I lost much of
the strength and feeling in my legs and feet. I was no longer able
to run, nor even wiggle my toes.

**the time that Aunt Mary called us in the middle of the night
     to tell us that Muehlstein Rubber Company, the
     Jersey City factory where my father worked, was
     burning to the ground**
and how we were able to see the flames from our apartment
          window a mile or so away

**my mother telling me that she worked at the Dixon
     Ticonderoga Company pencil factory in Jersey City
     when she was young**
- Years later, the Dixon buildings were renovated into a
residential apartment complex and Nadine and I were one of its
first tenants. When we took my mother to see the apartment, she
remarked that she could still smell the lead from the pencils.

loving to bowl as a teenager
and having my own bowling ball, bag, and shoes
and once calling my father from a pay telephone to tell him that I
          just rolled three strikes in a row - a turkey!
and the time I actually beat my father (89 to 88), although he had
          a huge sty on his eye and could hardly see

- Although I only took a step or two before releasing the ball, I found this more difficult to do as I got older and was forced to cut short this budding sports career.

playing chess in High School
- I later joined the United States Chess Federation and played in several tournaments (and actually won one). I would have arguments with a fellow attorney who contended that chess was not a "sport." This was my last chance to be an "athlete!"

buying one share of stock at around twelve years old (Wheeling Steel) from a stockbroker on Journal Square
and learning that the stockbroker was Johnny Kucks, the New York Yankee pitcher who won the seventh game of the 1956 World Series against the Brooklyn Dodgers
and learning that my brother Morris knew Johnny Kucks
and remembering that I had gotten a baseball autographed by Kucks at a neighborhood Christmas party hosted by my brothers' friend Willie Wolfe
and Wheeling Steel not being a very good investment for me, as over the next several months, I spent about as much money buying the New York Times each day, to check the stock, as I paid for the stock itself

Mrs. Voltz, her brother Louie, and her son Howard living in the apartment directly under ours
and the time Mrs. Voltz painted her toilet bowl black and her toilet seat silver
and their not having a TV
and Mrs. Voltz coming up to our apartment every now and then to watch our TV

and how in the summer, our window fan brought Louie's cigar
       smoke into our apartment

**playing Santa Claus as an eighth grader in the Christmas
       play at A. Harry Moore**
and except for Mrs. Claus, all the other parts being played by
       third and fourth-graders
and singing a song in the show
- While in law school, I took a few acting lessons at the HB
Studio in New York City. As an adult, I also landed parts in two
shows produced by small theater groups; however, on both
occasions, I quit shortly after beginning.

being in the A. Harry Moore School Choir
and singing the Cantata, "Song of Hiawatha," or at least part of
      it, at our only concert

my mother picking up Playboy Magazine for me each month
and my friends coming to my house to read it (well, perhaps not
      to "read" it)

taking Mechanical Dentistry at A. Harry Moore
and thinking about being a dental technician
- After quitting high school, I did apply for a job as a dental
technician. I was rejected because they were looking for someone
with experience. I do, however, have a half pair of dentures (the
uppers) in my memorabilia box.

**arguing with Kenny Smith in the auditorium prior to the
start of class one morning**
and Kenny asking me if I wanted to fight (He was a year ahead of
me and in much better shape)
and my agreeing to fight because there were a lot of kids around
and he and I going to the lavatory
and my being punched squarely in the nose before I knew what
happened
and walking back into the auditorium holding my nose
- I thought that I might as well try to get a laugh out of an
embarrassing situation. I was successful.

**Tessa being very heavy and having a difficult time walking
due to Muscular Dystrophy**
and my joking with her now and then, by very lightly "punching"
her on the arm
and our teacher one day pulling me aside and telling me not to do
that anymore because Tessa was getting weaker and it
could cause her to fall

**Donald being overheard one day by a teacher, as he was
saying something about not going to church**
and the teacher remarking that he should go to church to stay in
God's good graces
and Donald becoming teary-eyed and asking the teacher, "Where
was God and His good graces when I lost my leg?"

Ricky and Guido doing "steps" on the bandstand
and my being embarrassed because I was unable to join them

playing cards on the Staten Island Ferry
and enjoying the gentle soothing nature of the water
and staying on the boat over and over again, until being thrown
        off by the attendant
- I didn't need sea sickness patches back then, but did need them
when Nadine and I later cruised Alaska's Inside Passage. The
highlight of our trip was a walk on the Mendenhall Glacier (with
the aid of a helicopter to get there and moon boots to keep from
slipping on the ice).

driving Pierre, our "soap-box" car

always talking about how I wanted to parachute jump
and people telling me that my legs wouldn't be strong enough to
        land safely
- Although I never jumped, I did have introductory flights in a
small plane and a glider (a plane without an engine). In each
case, I was given control of the craft for a minute or so. My
friend Al took flying lessons for a few months (in a Piper
Cherokee) and actually soloed twice. He gave it up shortly after
meeting his wife-to-be.

**my mother getting mad because I took the training wheels off
        my bike**
and her giving me one chance to ride it without falling
and going just a few feet before I fell
and the bike being put away for the rest of the summer
- My brother Morris was there and offered to put the training
wheels back on the bike, but my mother wouldn't hear of it.

riding in the trunk of Peter and Louie's car (They were twins)
and then two of my friends getting in the trunk to ride together
- I think this was about the time of the Gemini space flights.

digging to China
- I guess so I could get all the tea that was there.

my mother making "brains"
and eating and loving them until I was old enough to understand
that they really were "brains"
- My mother used to coat the lamb brains in egg and bread
crumbs and fry them in oil. Anyone for some Rocky Mountain
oysters?

my parents living most of their youth on or around Center Street, in the mostly Italian downtown area of Jersey City
- I took my mother and my Aunt Tessie to that area years later.
They pointed out where their house used to be. The Eastern
Extension of the New Jersey Turnpike has replaced it.

Factory Street in Jersey City, where my grandmother and other relatives lived
- It's also gone.

going shopping with my mother on "the Avenue" (Central Avenue)
and John's Bargain Store
and Cheap Sam's

and the Acme being the first supermarket to have air
        conditioning
and my mother, more often than not, on our way home, buying
        me a five-cent cupcake at Goehrig's Bakery
and the cupcake being fully devoured well before reaching home
        (although traces of it would surely remain)

**going to the Central Theater on Central Avenue by Bus to
        meet my friends who walked there**
and getting sixty cents from my mother for the movie, bus fare,
        and goodies
- The Central is long gone.

**going by myself to the State Theater on Journal Square when
        I got a little older to see "House on Haunted Hill" with
        Vincent Price**
and my mother making me two baloney sandwiches to take with
        me
and the movie being done in a new technique (I forget what it
        was called)
and near the end of the movie, the screen darkening, and a
        skeleton coming out of a box that was on stage
and the skeleton sailing over the heads of the audience (on some
        sort of cable)
and nearly dropping one of my baloney sandwiches (I did say
        nearly)
- Coincidentally, on the day I am editing this recollection, I read
in a local newspaper that the State Theater was recently
demolished.

Note: A search on the internet reveals that the "skeleton"
technique was called "Emergo," a gimmick that apparently made
the film a huge success.

51

going to the "Café Wha?" in New York's Greenwich Village with James Elieff on Thanksgiving Eve in 1963

going to 42nd Street in Manhattan with Bruce, to try to get into a "dirty" movie

and Bruce having phoney "proof"

and my changing my birth certificate to read 1945 instead of 1948

and showing it to the manager of the theater

and the manager asking me why I didn't have a draft card since I was eighteen years old

and my answering that I was handicapped and couldn't go into the army

and the manager arguing that I would still have a draft card, but would be classified "4F"

and Bruce taking the manager aside to talk to him (probably giving him a sad story about this poor crippled kid just wanting to see some tits)

and finally being let into the theater

and sitting down (in the midst of mostly "old" guys) to watch a nudist film

and the most exciting scene consisting of a few young women playing volley ball

- A few years later, I learned that the theater manager was correct. I had received a letter ordering me to report to the local office of the Selective Service System on Journal Square. Shortly thereafter, I was sent a draft card with the classification "4F."

Mr. Look (a very elderly man with a thick German accent)

and his yelling at kids when they went on or near his property

and how he once called me a "crippled bastard" in front of my friends

- I generally cringe when I hear the term "crippled." It has such a pejorative connotation. As an adult, I once sent a letter of complaint to newspaper columnist Kay Gardella for her use of the word "crippled" in describing a disabled person in a TV movie. She did not respond to my letter.

Note: I recently received an email from a fellow alumnus of the A. Harry Moore School, Vincent Ferraro, who has begun a website about the school, its alumni, faculty, and staff (www.aharrymoore.org). There are pictures on the site also. I was very surprised to see in one of the pictures that apparently the school was first named: A. Harry Moore School for Crippled Children. Of course, that was 1931.

children saying to their mother or father, "Look at the way that kid walks"
- Not too many years later it would be, "Look at the way that fat man walks." The parent's response would run the gamut from no acknowledgment, to chastising the child. Most often it would be a look of embarrassment. Although I felt no anger toward the child or parent, it did make me extremely uncomfortable. Except for "Jerry's Kids" and the annual Cerebral Palsy Telethon "Look at Us We're Walking" parade around Dennis James and Jane Pickens Langley, there was not much exposure for the disabled back then. Moreover, quite often, the limited exposure that did exist portrayed the disabled as a somewhat pathetic lot. Although this attitude toward the disabled has certainly been changing in recent years, there is much more to be accomplished. I once saw Itzak Perlman walking through a record shop in New York City. I was excited because I saw a world renowned violinist. I was not sad because I saw a man walking with crutches.

having someone open or hold open a door for me
- Although I understood the gesture as basically one of kindness,

there was always an undercurrent of negativity associated with it. Today when this happens, I will try to get to the next door first so that I can return the favor. Of course, I usually don't make it.

looking through a Sears & Roebuck catalog and remarking that I would like to buy ski equipment

and my aunt and cousin telling me that I wouldn't be able to ski
- I believed that, for the next thirty-three years, until I skied down the beginner's slope (not the bunny slope) at Ski Windham in New York. Although I was taking part in a program for disabled skiers, it was truly an exhilarating experience.

my friends and I watching stag films in my kitchen as my mother and father watched TV in the living room

and placing the movie screen in front of the door connecting the kitchen to the living room, so that we would have to move the screen to let my mother or father into the kitchen and, therefore, have reason to stop the projector and Ricky saying each time my father walked into the room,
"What do you say guys, want to watch the fights again?"
- I did have an 8mm film featuring great boxing matches, but I think Ricky overdid it a bit.

being seventeen and going to my first all night party at a friend's house

and during the early evening, one of the girls getting very drunk and various guys trying to take advantage of her and one of her girlfriends bringing her over to sit with me and saying, "You stay here, you'll be safe with Carmine" and not feeling very complimented by that statement and in the early morning hours, being very hungry and several of us getting in a car to go looking for food

and grabbing a bag of recently delivered bread, which just
        happened to be sitting innocently in front of a yet-to-open
        grocery store
and eating some of it, then bringing the rest back
and leaving a note with the bread:

        Thank you for the bread. It was delicious.
        (Signed) BLOW (Bread Lovers of Wisconsin)

**four of us playing ball in front of Gallagher's Tavern with a
        real baseball bat (Gallagher's occupied the ground
        floor of the apartment building where I lived)**
and Ray losing his grip on the bat as he swung
and the bat going through Gallagher's large window
and all of us running in different directions
and several weeks later, each of our parents getting a letter in the
        mail from Gallagher's lawyer or insurance carrier asking
        for $51.00 (one-quarter of the cost of the window)
and not being sure how Gallagher found out who was involved
- As far as I know, no one ever paid the claim, and we never heard
anything more about it.

**Gallagher, the tavern owner, ringing our bell and yelling,
        "Scarpa - phone call!"**
- This, of course, was before we had our first telephone.

**my father putting a lobster between me and the back of my
        wheelchair (I was just home from the hospital)**
and our next-door neighbor telling me that she almost called the
        police when she heard me screaming
- Although my father meant it as a joke, I couldn't comfortably
look at a lobster again until nearly thirty years later when, at

Nadine's urging, I tried it (and loved it) at a Portuguese restaurant in the Ironbound section of Newark. I, in turn, introduced Nadine to the exquisite nature of garlic.

John bringing a Bob Dylan album to my house
and how we laughed at the sound of his voice and thought that
        Dylan was an old man
and how I purchased a Hohner harmonica with an around-the-
        neck holder that very next week

going to New York with my guitar in hand and playing some
        of my original compositions for Russ Vincent of Kama
        Sutra Records
and his being interested in one of my songs, saying that it would
        be a good tune for Percy Sledge to record
and his passing on the song when I called him back a couple of
        days later

going to see The Beatles at Shea Stadium in 1965 with James
        Elieff instead of playing the "Casino" at Palisade
        Amusement Park with my band
- Years later, John and I would go for pizza at Patsy's in Brooklyn with Sid Bernstein, the promoter of that first-ever ballpark concert. Talk about "six degrees of separation." John had met him at a song writers' class and they became friends. A year or so later, Sid invited me to a concert he was promoting at the French Alliance in New York City featuring Genette Reno, a French-Canadian singer. Nadine was with me, and when I introduced her to Sid, he, being ever the gentleman, said, "Nadine, your reputation precedes you." I quickly looked at Nadine and said, "Don't blame me. I didn't say a thing."

**going with James to see the premiere showing of The Beatles'
   first movie, "A Hard Day's Night" at the Loew's
   Theater in Newark**
and wondering how I was going to be able to run away from the
   screaming throngs of girls when I became famous

**going to Atlantic City to audition for Tony Grant's
   Steel Pier Show**
and Guido (our lead guitarist) seeing a sign on the highway that
   read: "Deer Crossing"
and Guido asking John's father, "Hey, Mr. Thiel, how do the deer
   know where to cross?"

**becoming a bass player since there were three guitars in our
   first rock band and I was the last one in**
and the other band members teasing me by saying that I thought I
   was Paul McCartney
- John Lennon later became my favorite Beatle.

**the band appearing on Sonny Fox's "Just for Fun" television
   show on Channel 5 in New York**
and doing a song called "Topo Gigio" which Ricky and I wrote
   about Ed Sullivan's Italian mouse
and thinking that Ed would see us and invite us on his show
and that not happening
and how Ed, about a month later, introduced two members of his
   orchestra who played an instrumental tune called "Topo
   Gigio"
and the duo ending their song the same way we ended ours, with
   the catch phrase,"Eddie, kiss me goodnight"
- Ed may not have seen our performance, but you couldn't
convince us that these two orchestra members hadn't.

John's Aunt Dorothy
and how she was a famous clairvoyant
and Aunt Dorothy telling us that she knew Ed Sullivan and, if we
　　　fired our manager, she would get our band on the show
- We didn't. She didn't. We had lost a second chance to be on the
Ed Sullivan Show.

**the orchestra leader for the Ed Sullivan and Jackie Gleason
　　　television shows being Ray Bloch**
and Jackie introducing him as "the flower of the music world"
and Jackie later using Sammy Spear

**the band playing on a live television show on channel 47
　　　in Newark**
and the show being hosted by John Zacharly (the same "Zacharly"
　　　who years earlier had hosted monster movies on TV)
and our band, at the time, featuring a five-year-old girl who played
　　　organ
and thinking that this novelty would be our ticket to the big time
- I guess there are not too many short cuts to the big time.

**listening to "I Wish That We Were Married" (by Ronnie and
　　　the Hi-Lites) on the radio**
- It would be a great thrill to later meet and become friends with
Ronnie (through John), and to play behind Ronnie as he sang that
song during a jam session in John's living room. It would be very
sad to go to Ronnie's wake just a few short years after that.

**John's Uncle Rocky taking us to play for military veterans at
　　　a hospital in the Bronx**
and how some amputees applauded by hitting their remaining

hand against their chest
- Rocky was a comedian and went by the name of Tony Stevens.
He died just a few months before I edited this recollection.

my parents reading the newspaper obituaries each day
- My doing the same today.

**staying at A. Harry Moore for the first half of my freshman
      year of high school**
and Mrs. Pollack being a young and beautiful teacher
and how Jeffrey, who had a rather severe case of Cerebral Palsy,
      used to fall on the floor in front of her in an attempt to
      look up her dress
- Looking back, I think that Jeffrey may have told us that to give
an alternate reason for his frequent falling.

**Mrs. Pollack getting mad at me one day during class and
      making me stand in the corner for a few minutes**
and this being quite embarrassing
and it also being slightly arousing

**deciding to transfer to Dickinson High School (the "normal"
      school) for the second half of freshman year**
and saying very proudly to the kids in the neighborhood, "Hey, I
      go to Dickinson"
and their replying to me, "Yea, so? We all do"

the one-way halls at Dickinson
and barely making it to my next class before the bell

the Dickinson football coach pinching my chubby cheek and
   saying, "Why don't you come out for the team?"
- He had yet to see me walking the halls.

singing "Don't Let the Sun Catch You Crying" with my
   band at the Friday Auditorium show at Dickinson
and playing the school dance that afternoon

being taught by an eighth grader (when I was in fifth) how to
   train my hair for that "pompadour" look
and wearing one of my mother's old stockings over my head each
   night when I went to bed

James Elieff and I going to Snyder High School (out of our
   district) because we got transportation supplied by the
   A. Harry Moore school bus and because Snyder had an
   elevator
and James once carrying a package of French cigarettes (De
   Murier)
and he and I telling an A. Harry Moore student that it was
   marijuana
and the next day my being called out of English class and down to
   the Vice Principal's office
and the Vice Principal sitting me down, looking at me very
   seriously, and asking, "What do you know about
   Marijuana?"
and immediately realizing the source of this inquiry and telling
   him the story
and James later telling me that two men took him out of class and
   searched his locker without telling him why

James having a heart condition that left him very frail
and his hands being very knobby
and his fingernails being blue
and a couple of students calling him "Buzz" (for buzzard, I guess)
       and teasing him during lunch times
and my taking these guys aside one day and telling them that
       James was a karate expert and that his hands looked as
       they did because he used them to break wooden boards
       and bricks
and James no longer being bothered by these students
and James later having corrective surgery

riding the school bus with Richie Wright
and Richie being a dwarf (a little person)
and asking Richie (for whatever reason, I don't know) why he was
       transported to Snyder High by the A. Harry Moore
       school bus
and Richie shrugging his shoulders and answering,
       "I don't know"

going to Snyder baseball games at the "old high school field"
and hoping that Anthony Calabrese, the celebrated Snyder hurler,
       would be starting that day

wiping up Ricky's vomit from my kitchen floor while my
       mother and father were asleep
- He had just had an argument with his girlfriend and had been
slugging down Four Roses whiskey. I had to walk him home
before cleaning up the mess. I was happy to discover that neither
of my parents got up to go to the bathroom while I was gone. They
would have walked right through it.

Aunt Raffie (Raffaella) telling me about Melfi, the town in southern Italy where she was born and where my maternal ancestors originated
and how the town was in the hills and had a wall around it
and how she came to Ellis Island at age twelve

my cousin Vinnie (The real one!) playing trumpet with his band, at my cousin (his brother) Anthony's wedding in Bayonne, New Jersey
- I remember it being a "football wedding" with large tables filled with wrapped sandwiches. I think the term comes from people "tossing" sandwiches to one another. During Connie's wedding in the "Godfather," as one of the guests is tossing sandwiches to Paulie, he shouts, "Hey, Paulie, I got two gabagool! Gabagool!" His pronunciation of "capicola" (Italian hot ham) is based on a southern Italian dialect used quite often by Italian-Americans. As a kid, I always said, "manigut" (for manicotti), "ganool" (for canolli) and, of course, "goomba" (for compari). My father and my Uncle Al shortened "goomba" even further and called each other "goomp."

listening to tape recordings of my father singing with Joe Small accompanying him on the accordion (or piano)
- There are only a few seconds of those tapes left. They were either lost or inadvertently erased. A prime example of youth taking things for granted.

my father singing "I Wonder What's Become of Sally" at family functions
and my band once playing behind him, but not doing such a good job since I was the only band member that had ever heard the song (and even I didn't know the chords)

- Shortly after my father's death, I called in to the Jonathan
Schwartz Radio Show to ask him if he knew the song (Jonathan
was a radio DJ and a Sinatra "aficionado"). He not only said
"yes," but named the composer (Milton Ager) and the lyricist
(Jack Yellin). The song was written in 1924 and was sung by Al
Jolson. Years later, I would have dinner with Jonathan Schwartz
at a "Sinatra Round Table." I had been one of seven winners of a
radio contest where the contestants had to sing the next line of a
Sinatra song. My song was "All the Way." It was a privilege to
have sung a "duet" with Sinatra. My father would have enjoyed
that.

**my father being reluctant or unable to express his feelings for
        his family**
- At his wake, I was surprised and greatly comforted when two of
his longtime friends told me how he used to brag about me and
my music. They said that everything was ". . . my kid this and my
kid that . . . " I knew my father liked the fact that I was in a band,
that I was the lead ballad singer and that I sang many standard
songs, especially Sinatra. He used to bring my mother and my
Aunt Mary to hear us when we played at local nightclubs. About
six years after his death, the last bass guitar he purchased for me
was stolen out of the trunk of my car, as I studied for the bar exam
at Town Hall in New York City. I never replaced it. After playing
for a while with a borrowed bass, I stopped playing altogether.

**how Aunt Glady and Uncle Frank once lived near Sinatra in
        Hoboken, New Jersey**
and my using their "shared" bathroom (No, they didn't share it
        with Sinatra but with the family in the apartment next
        door)
and the bathroom having two doors, one for each family
and how upon entering the chamber, you would fasten a chain

across the width of the room so that it hung taut between the two doors, making it impossible to open either door from the outside

- Standing up in a hurry could have snapped your head off. Why this procedure, rather than a hook and eye or some similar locking device? Presumably, because to exit the bathroom you had no choice but to unfasten the chain. If a hook and eye were used, you might forget to unlock the other family's door. Besides being an unneighborly thing to do, such an omission could potentially cause much distress.

always wanting to play my cousin Sal's guitar

my father not allowing Aunt Tessie and Uncle Al to buy me a bicycle as a gift for my grammar school graduation
and his expressing a strong fear that bicycles were too dangerous in the city
and his having no such fear years before, when Aunt Tessie and Uncle Al bought bicycles for my brothers upon their graduations

wanting a paper route
and my mother and father being firmly against it
and upon their refusing to give me the five dollars needed for a bond, my threatening to go out to shine shoes for the money
and the threat not changing their minds
and leaving the apartment with shoe shine kit in hand

- They didn't think I could handle the paper route since I didn't like walking long distances. Apparently, for the same reason, they were not very worried about the prospect of me actually going out to shine shoes. Having not gone more than two inches outside the apartment, and with my ear hard-pressed against the door, I heard my father say, "I have a mind to give him the five dollars just to prove to him that he can't do it." I immediately reentered the apartment. The next day I changed my mind about taking the job.

my father and his friends singing the song "Wop"

> Hey wop! Hey wop! Hey wop!
> I wonder why they call me wop.
> Why it's just the biggest shame,
> How they call me nickie names.
> They shouted Tony, you're so phoney,
> You look just like a macaroni.
> Guinea! Dago! Wop!
> I wish the cop would make them stop.
> First they called me Dago,
> Then it's guinea, guinea, guinea.
> Now it's wop.
> Hey wop!
> Shut up!

- For those who don't know, the term "wop" (used disparagingly against Italian-Americans) was derived from immigrants coming to America "without papers." I don't know who wrote this song, but I suppose it typified the kind of treatment many newly arrived European ethnic groups received. As it turned out, I was the first professional in our immediate family and I am saddened that my father died before seeing me go to law school. Although his initial reaction may have been to doubt the likelihood of my success, I think he would have been happy with the outcome. I should also note that coming along much later than my brothers allowed me certain privileges and advantages that, unfortunately, my brothers did not have.

**playing the stereo while watching the neighborhood goings-on
from my fire escape window**
and quickly ducking inside if I saw friends approaching since I
didn't want them to know that I had nothing better to do

**being quite sedentary in my teens due to my disability and
growing obesity**

being child-cruel to Linda
and how no one had ever seen Linda's mother
and Linda telling everyone that her mother was in the hospital
and my blurting out one day, "Your mother's not in the hospital.
That's what they tell kids when their mother is dead"
and Linda crying
- I will never forget her face. I will also never forget the day that
Linda's mother returned from the hospital. I have heard it said that
a person with a clear conscience probably has a bad memory.

becoming a Junior Deputy Sheriff
and going to a half-day event where a judge spoke to us in his
courtroom
and then being taken through an underground tunnel which
connected the courthouse and the jail
and being locked in a cell for a minute or so
and being given a nice shiny badge to pin in my wallet
and threatening kids in my neighborhood with arrest if they didn't
listen to me
- It was very interesting to later see that courthouse again when I
returned there as an attorney.

playing "Cowboys and Indians" with the two black kids living
next door to my Aunt Tessie and Uncle Al (They were
the cowboys and I was the Indian)

how Aunt Tessie and Uncle Al moved to Florida shortly after
the 1968 riots in their predominately black Jersey City
neighborhood

listening to the radio in my fifth-grade classroom as Allen
Shepherd became the first "Man in Space"
and being very surprised when he came down so fast

being called Pontius Pilate by a guy from the South Street
Gang

having others "run for me" when playing baseball or stickball

Jimmy Beam doing a play by play of our games in his Phil
Rizzuto voice

my first 45 RPM being Elvis' "Heartbreak Hotel"
and my second 45 RPM being Elvis' "Hound Dog"
and my first LP being Elvis' "Elvis"
and my second LP being Elvis' "Loving You"

abandoning Elvis for Jerry Lee Lewis (ever so briefly)
and my mother crocheting a hair piece for me to use, so I could
make my hair fall over my eyes when I shook my head like

Jerry Lee.

abandoning Mickey Mantle for Roger Maris

**walking on the field in Yankee Stadium (They used to let you
        do that after a game)**
and picking up some centerfield grass
and taping it into my Yankee Yearbook with the notation: "Grass
        that Mickey Mantle stepped on"

**John and I drinking liquor from the bottles in his parents'
        liquor cabinet**
and John's mother getting suspicious and marking the fluid levels
        on the bottles
and getting caught and having John's mother tell my mother
and all the liquor bottles in my house having rings of nail polish
        around them
- Didn't they know that you could replace one liquid with
another? Anyone for Chivas Regal "Light"?

the first time I met John
and how, for Lord knows what reason, I asked him if he wanted to
        fight
and John and I rolling around on the ground
and my mother yelling from the window above, "You leave
        Carmine alone" (She actually said, "Carmen." All my
        friends and family pronounced my name that way)
and this same scenario happening a few times
- Years later, John would feel vindicated when my mother and
Aunt Tessie finally learned (from John - who else?) that I was the
instigator of those fights. Oh well, boys will be boys.

John and I becoming friends because we both played accordion

and becoming an accordion duo called "The Royals"

and having our first (and only) gig at the Jersey City Women's Club

and getting paid one dollar each (and all the fancy colored fishcakes we could eat)

- Ick!

my father's nicknames being "Nooch," "Noochie," and "Noochie Molly"

- I think it was based on the Italian, "Carminooch." Molly was his mother's name. I have been called "Carminooch" quite often also.

my mother and father playing 500 Rummy

and my father winning more often than not

and, on those occasions when my mother did manage to win, his slamming the cards down on the table and yelling, "You don't know how to play the game"

and my mother's quiet smile

writing many poems throughout school

and some being downright autobiographical:

> Slow the fat bear moves
> He eats his macaroni
> He says its diet gravy
> It's not, he's just a phoney

the pony rides at Bergen Point Amusement Park (a.k.a. Uncle Miltie's) in Bayonne

and my parents taking me there about once a year when we visited
Aunt Raffie and Uncle Tony at their bakery

and the time I was next in line to get on a pony (probably after
devouring a canolli and an éclair at the bakery)

and the petite little girl waiting behind me

and the next pony prancing alongside the raised platform on
which we were waiting being a small frilly one

and lifting my leg toward the pony in preparation to get on

and the man operating the ride yelling, "Hey, wait, this pony is too
small for you"

and my father quickly adding, "Yea, what do you want to do, kill
that pony?"

and watching in silence as the little girl got on that pony and rode
away

and waiting patiently as the next beast of burden, a large
unadorned nag, hobbled up to the platform

Mrs. Burkholtz and her husband Tony living next to us after Josephine and her family left

and how Tony, at age ninety-two, used to tell me stories about
"old" Jersey City (He was born just a few years after the
Civil War ended)

and the time I played a song from one of my accordion books,
while Tony sang the song's German lyrics to his wife

and how Mrs. Burkholtz cried

- Remembering the past can evoke warmth.

saying "Nigger Babies" instead of "Chocolate Babies" at the candy store

- Remembering the past can also summon regret.

making Eddie Burke cry by calling him "nigger" at school
- As a young adult, I would write a play in which the underlying
theme was the evil of racism. John chose and directed the play for
a Christian Youth Organization (C.Y.O.) play competition. I was
additionally flattered when the Drama Club at William Paterson
College produced my play called "Raca" (a Hebrew/Aramaic
word meaning "fool").

"The Bitter End" (an 8mm film I made with James Elieff)
and having it shown during an open screening night at
        Filmmaker's Cinematheque in New York City
- This was the theater famous for showing "underground films"
and, in particular, for showing the early works of Andy Warhol,
including "Empire," an eight-hour long single view of the Empire
State Building (from dark 'till dawn). Our film was conceived and
made as a serious message film about drugs and it received
probably the best audience response of any film shown that
evening. The downside, however, was that the audience thought
that our film was a comedy. Well, one of the purposes of art is to
entertain, isn't it?

**Linda and I having a contest to see who would go farther into
        the street (something we were not allowed to do)**
and Howard (Mrs. Voltz's adult son) standing near us
and my being aware that Howard was not looking our way
and Linda and I taking turns going progressively farther into the
        street, until I finally summoned the nerve to go all the way
and Linda running to tell my mother what I had done
and my mother (who had been sitting on the front stoop) slapping
        me a few times on my arms (It was one of the rare times
        that I was hit by either of my parents)
and feeling very angry with my mother and Linda
and seeing Howard walking toward us and saying to my mother,

"Howard was with us, he'll tell you that I didn't go into the street"
- Of course, Howard supported my version of what had happened since he hadn't seen me cross the street. Although my mother didn't apologize to me, I could tell she was sorry. She also yelled at Linda for "lying." This is not an episode I am happy about recounting.

playing third base on crutches with a cast on my leg

playing quarterback against the Van Nostrand Avenue team (I had a very good throwing arm)
and our opposition being coached by my schoolmate, John Seccafico (from his wheelchair)
and John not letting any of his players tackle me
and our still losing 44 to 0 when the game was called at half-time
and expressing our anger over the game being called early
and John's father giving us money for a taxi home (He had been the referee)
- That's it. The fix was in.

going into Sandy's pool with a T-shirt (my breasts being larger than most of the girls in the neighborhood)
and socks (my feet having surgical scars)
and an automobile inner tube around my waist (not being able to swim - although the need not being readily apparent in a nine-foot diameter, three-foot deep pool)

the Washington Park ("North Street Park") Swimming Pool
and the time some kid let the air out of my inner tube

Mrs. Pizzelli
and how she would throw a bucket of water on us when she
      caught us sitting on her stoop

peeing in public places
- A symptom of my Spina Bifida is a neurogenic bladder - one
that does what it wants to, when it wants to. I was about thirty-six
when I learned that there were medications to control this
problem.

**peeing into the Hawaiian Punch can after coming home from
      the hospital**
and my mother (and sometimes my friends, if they were willing)
      bringing the can to me when I needed it

being on stage and having an uncontrollable urge to pee
and just putting down my guitar and walking off
and being embarrassed to go back on stage
- But I did.

**a few of us looking up "teat" in the dictionary in the ninth
      grade at A. Harry Moore**
and a girl looking at us with disdain and saying, "You're in High
      School now. Grow up!"
and feeling embarrassed as she wheeled herself out of the room

**my brother Ralph telling me that, before I was born, the
      owner of the local bakery would sometimes give my
      mother day-old bread for free**
and my mother saying to my father, "Hey, I think the bakery guy

likes me. He gives me day-old bread for free"
and my father remarking to my mother (jokingly, of course), "Tell
    the bakery guy that, if he gives us fresh bread, he can have
    you"

**Ralph telling me that he and Janet were going to have their
    first child**
and his explaining to me that I was going to be an uncle
and then adding, "That's if it's a boy. But if it's a girl, you'll be an
    aunt!"
- It was a girl.

my first kiss (with "Cookie" in the fifth-grade clothing room)
and how she told everyone that she had lost her leg while hitching
    a freight train in Hoboken (It's possible that she lost her
    leg in a less dramatic fashion, but then again, how less
    dramatically can a child lose a leg?)
and she and I pressing against each other one day on the crowded
    school elevator
and confessing to each other that evening on the telephone that we
    had found the experience very pleasurable
and further agreeing that we would kiss the next day in the
    clothing room
and it being several days, perhaps weeks, until we had the
    opportunity or, more accurately, the courage to meet in the
    clothing room, since both of us were extremely hesitant
    and shy about going through with our plan
and somehow, finally managing to get close enough so that our
    lips touched
and when it was over, backing up a bit and looking at each other
    as if to say, is that all there is? Did we do something
    wrong?
- As happens so often, the anticipation of an event is greater than

the event itself. We never really spoke about that kiss, but we did kiss again some twenty years later when we met by chance at a New Year's Eve Party at which Cookie was a guest and my band was playing. Although she appeared to be with a date, we did manage to say a few words to each other during the evening. Quite unexpectedly, however, at the stroke of midnight, while I was on the bandstand playing "Auld Lang Syne," Cookie came up to me and planted a long, hard, wet one. Cookie had lost her shyness, and I nearly lost my glasses. Although it took some twenty years, I think we finally shared a bit of that moment we thought we'd missed out on that day in the fifth-grade clothing room.

the day Lorraine was being examined by the school doctor
> **(We were all examined periodically so the school could assess our conditions)**

and how I watched from the waiting room through a partially
> opened door

and telling Lorraine that afternoon on the school bus that I had
> seen her in her panties (although I didn't really see much
> of anything)

and her asking me what color they were

and my guessing "pink"

and her answering "white"

and my feigning disbelief

and her saying that she would prove it to me

and my obvious exhilaration being short-lived as the school bus
> arrived at Lorraine's house

and that next morning when she got on the bus

and Lorraine coming over to me and whispering, "Come with me
> to the back of the bus and I'll show you my panties"

and how, in the back of the bus, away from prying eyes, and just
> as my anticipation was truly peaking (as much as it could
> in an eight-year-old): Lorraine showed me her white

panties.
- She had taken them out of her book bag.

hearing now and again about a woman having "woman trouble"

the whip
- No, this is not an S & M reference, but a children's ride that traveled throughout the city on a truck. The ride's cars would swiftly "whip" around the truck's short oval track. Not bad for a dime.

cruising up and down Park Avenue in Rutherford over and over again (à la "American Graffiti") in Sandy's car
- I don't recall which car Sandy had at that time, but I do remember when he got his brand new white Chrysler Cordoba - the one with red "Corinthian leather" (as Ricardo Montalban used to say in the television commercial).

my mother and Aunt Tessie telling me about the male boarder who lived in their house when they were teens
and how my grandmother, for financial reasons, had to take in a
    boarder once in a while
and how my mother and her sisters would take baths in a tub in
    the living area of the house
and how one day they observed an unusual movement in the
    curtain which separated the boarder's area from theirs
and how my grandmother, stick in hand, chased the boarder out of
    the house

a multitude of things about my mother
- However, since she passed away just a week before writing this paragraph, none of them seem important enough to act as tribute. Perhaps there is something too final about a tribute. I remembered my father's last words to me as he lay dying in the hospital emergency room, "Take care of your mother." Well, I did my best, Dad. I can also hear him saying, "Don't worry. Your mother and I have seats by the drummer." And it's funny, but I'm starting to sense more clearly the nature of that drummer.

John Dunwoodie and Eddie Burke
and being close friends at A. Harry Moore
and mimicking "The Three Stooges" (John played Moe, Eddie
          played Larry, and I, of course, played Curley)
and our being pretty good
and Eddie having a pronounced limp (perhaps from polio)
and never being certain why John was at A. Harry Moore since he
          had no obvious disability
- It was not very common for kids to talk about their disabilities. Whatever John's problem, however, it must have resolved, since just a few minutes before editing this recollection, I learned that he had been highly decorated for his service in the Vietnam War. He had, among other decorations, won the bronze star. I learned this information from his obituary in the newspaper. John had died at age forty-four, leaving behind a wife and three children.

Note: I recently received an email from John Dunwoodie's wife who said that her son was doing an internet search of his father's name when he came across my fine art photography website on which I had posted some of these childhood memories. She said that her son was very happy to see this recollection about his father. She also said in her email that John had gone to A. Harry Moore due to his having asthma and that his condition eventually did resolve.

John Seccafico

and he being my closest friend at A. Harry Moore (He had polio
       and would always be confined to a wheelchair)
and talking with John all day at school and then half the evening
       on the telephone at home
and that day in the fourth grade when John was being transferred
       to another class (he was a half-year ahead of me)
and both of us crying like babies
and making such a scene that teachers from other rooms (perhaps
       other floors) came to watch
- About twenty years or so after school, I ran into John at a
wedding at which my band was playing. We could only speak for
a few minutes because I was working and he was with his family,
but we did exchange telephone numbers and promised each other
that we would get in touch during the coming week and arrange a
time and place for us to meet and talk over "old times." I thought
to myself, how great it will be to rekindle such a close friendship.
He never called me and I never called him.

      . . . perhaps when it comes to our memories, we are
ultimately afraid of subjecting our certain, though often sad past,
to our uncertain, though often happy present. Then again, to
borrow a phrase used by my father, perhaps that's just "donkey
dust."

About the Author

Carmine J. Scarpa is a municipal attorney residing in Jersey City, New Jersey. Prior to becoming an attorney, he was employed as a commercial artist and performed as a musician and vocalist.

Since graduating from law school in 1983, Mr. Scarpa's artistic endeavors have become increasingly important to him. In 2001, he received the H. Juergen Thieck Memorial Award for Photography from the Visual Arts Center of New Jersey.

Mr. Scarpa's fine art photography, as well as some of his paintings, conceptual art, and poetry, can be viewed on the web at Carmine Scarpa Galleries (www.carminescarpa.com).